W9-ANR-619

HOW TO IMPROVE YOUR POSTURE

Fran Lehen

Photographs by Fred Eberstadt

Drawings by Wendy Grossman

Cornerstone Library
Published by Simon & Schuster
New York

**Because of
Jeanne, Gail, and Jenny**

Copyright © 1982 by Fran Lehen

All rights reserved
including the right of reproduction
in whole or in part in any form
Published by Cornerstone Library
A Simon & Schuster Division of
Gulf & Western Corporation
Simon & Schuster Building
1230 Avenue of the Americas
New York, New York 10020

Designed by Leonard Telesca

CORNERSTONE LIBRARY and colophon are trademarks of
Simon & Schuster, registered in the U.S. Patent and Trademark Office.

First Cornerstone Library printing October 1982

10 9 8 7 6 5 4 3 2

Manufactured in the United States of America

Printed and bound by Semline, Inc.

ISBN: 0-346-12513-8

Contents

About the Author

Fran Lehen operates her own studio where she and her teachers teach the Pilates system of exercise.

She received her Pilates training from her teacher and mentor, Carola Trier, and taught at Mrs. Trier's studio for a number of years before opening her own. She is a licensed masseuse, having studied at the Swedish Institute of Massage in New York.

Her expertise is woven from her personal experience in learning to use her own body effectively and efficiently in order to pursue her interests in dance, self-defense, and gymnastics.

Ms. Lehen is a partner of SHAPE/TAPES, a firm producing exercise tapes.

Preface

Postural problems are as numerous as there are people to have them. Realizing that one small manual could not be helpful to all people, I had to make some very specific choices if I wanted to be helpful to some of them. The questions I thought needed answers were: What are the most common postural problems, and what approach would be most effective in a book of this nature?

What has surprised me the most in teaching my students is how little sensation, other than tightness or discomfort, they associate with certain areas of their anatomy. While trying to teach them exercises to stretch and strengthen these areas, I have felt that something was missing in their perception of their bodies. In order to get them to perform the exercises as I saw them, I realized an intermediate step was needed. That step was simply for them to gain a fuller awareness of their bodies. Before change can take place, an awakening has to happen.

My decision for the thrust of this book then, was to go for that awakening—what is involved to make it happen and how an individual can make it happen for himself. I chose to zero in on the areas of the body that can be awakened more readily and that the student feels more comfortable practicing away from the eye of a teacher. Included are exercises to sensitize the hands to enable them to help you sense your skeletal structure. There are also exercises to awaken and strengthen the feet to allow them to handle their weight bearing more efficiently. However, the main emphasis of the exercises in this book is on the spine, the shoulder girdle, and on the breath.

I don't presume to suggest that this manual can help all postural problems, even in the specific areas I've chosen to concentrate on, as the body can have deviations which require an expert working closely with that body in order to help make changes. But because of the concepts concerning learning I'm trying to communicate, I do feel this book can be helpful as a solid, basic start for a wide audience.

—Fran Lehen

Introduction

This book is designed to help you improve your posture. Naturally, included are a series of exercises to teach you about your body and its alignment. Since I believe good posture is more than holding your shoulders back and down, keeping your tummy in, and all the rest of the postural clichés and myths that have been heaped upon us, I feel it is essential for you to investigate your own myths and objectives to insure your success in this undertaking. So prepare yourselves; we have a lot of ground to cover before we get to the exercises.

POSTURE: GOOD OR OTHERWISE

Posture, according to the definition in my edition of Webster's New Collegiate Dictionary, is:

1. A relative arrangement of the different parts
2. Characteristic or assumed bearing; specifically pose of a model or figure
3. Condition, with reference to attitude
4. State or frame of mind

Definitions 3 and 4 may be a surprise to some people, but they are what underlies 1 and 2. Your posture is a

9

dead giveaway of where you are mentally as well as physically in your life. If this is the kind of statement you didn't expect in a posture improvement book, be prepared for a new learning venture for your body and mind. Before you can make a change in the relative arrangement of your body, you must examine its parts and your attitudes toward them.

After years of teaching and observing people, I've arrived at my own definition of posture, beginning with:

- posture is a state of being
- posture is your content
- posture is a way of life; an attitude
- posture is a statement to the world of your opinion of yourself, but good posture is a freedom . . . freedom from tension, from holding, and from tiredness and tightness. Good posture is giving up your misconceptions about posture, and permitting your body to do its job. Good posture, then, is a release from posturing. It's what we think of as "walking tall." Deciding to improve your posture is a decision to improve your life.

Chapter I

Self-knowledge

SELF-OBSERVATION

Most of us are intrigued with "people watching"—observing their behavior, clothes, and how they carry themselves. Almost without our conscious awareness, we pigeonhole them into categories: successful, aggressive, timid, or whatever fits our conclusion at that moment.

In the next few months, while working on your posture, shift your attention to yourself—become a "self-watcher"! If this seems like a bore or unnecessary, you're very much mistaken. It's imperative to know what you have to change or give up in order to let something else begin to happen. One way this can be accomplished is through thought. The only way you'll arrive at the proper "thought instruction" for yourself is through self-observation.

Self-observation can be difficult for some people although it is a way of life for others. Ideally, we should work toward the ability to use this faculty to help us in our endeavors (and not use it just in the name of vanity). Observe yourself consciously without judgment. Develop your inner sense of knowing how you're standing, sitting, or how your body is reacting to what is happening at the moment. Become conscious of how you sit while having coffee with your boss, for example. Did you sit differently when you had coffee with your friend? Did you feel tension in your upper back while having words with the cleaner for not having your trousers ready in time? When the bus pulled away just as you arrived at the corner, how long did it take you before you realized you were holding your shoulders up to your ears?

YOUR BODY NOTEBOOK

Wanting to improve your posture means changing your posture from something automatic, but evidently not satisfying, to something you haven't yet experienced. That's hard! Add to this the difficulty our thinking process has in focusing attention on something as "automatic" as our posture when faced with traffic, chores, scheduling our lives, and getting to work on time. It doesn't seem hard to understand why we let it go the way it is. However, our posture can be a nagging problem and what I am suggesting here is some structure to help you focus on these problematic habits.

When I'm working on a new level of personal growth or awareness, I have found it helpful to write down my thoughts. This way I begin to discover and understand what it is I actually think. A thought turned into the written word is not as fleeting as just "a thought." Once it's down on paper, I have a concrete place from which to start. It seems easier then, to move from one step to the next.

Get a small note pad. I say small, not because the subject matter is insignificant, but because it is easier to handle in a snatched moment, and can fit easily in a breast-coat pocket or pocketbook. To help you on your way I'm providing key questions which you can begin to answer in your notebook. Besides the notebook, all you will need to supply is a pencil and your concentration.

The keeping of this notebook may seem clumsy at first, but you'll get over this feeling. Don't censor your thoughts before you write them down. What we think are "silly observations" sometimes turn out to be important clues to how we need to change.

Here are some questions you may want to ask yourself:

1. What is your concept of good posture? Does it come from army exercise manuals or what you've always thought of as a feminine or masculine way to carry yourself? Whatever your concepts were or are, obviously at this point you're not pleased with them. Just acknowledge them now, and be ready to give some or all of them up.

There will be as many concepts of good posture as there are people writing them in their notebooks. That's the way it should be. We sometimes get confused and think there are "right" ways to perceive the world. We hide our own perceptions because we don't trust them; we're embarrassed that they may not be acceptable or, even worse, that they may be laughed at. It is true that we recognize beings of our species because of their upright position—a head centered on a stem in the middle of a width; an appendage hanging down each side of a trunk and two more standing on the earth. This is where the similarity ends and each member of the species becomes a separate entity. The number and position of appendages are no criteria for believing that what is good for one is necessarily good for two or all. Our likeness ends at the water line of the iceberg!

We're each a composite of our own experiences and our concepts will and should have our own unique stamp. Deep down inside every human being is an inner sense of what is appropriate and what is not appropriate for himself or herself, and I have respect for that inner resource.

In writing this manual, I will try to avoid generalizations. If I give an example, please realize that it is only an example, and that I'm aware of the millions of individual responses possible. The ideal would be a book on posture written with and for each person. Since that's out of the question, I've tried to make a gesture in that direction by guiding you in personalizing your own program.

In choosing a book on self-help (or an instructor in the flesh, for that matter), it is important not to completely suspend your expertise in personal selectivity and assume unequivocably that a teacher knows what's best for you. I suggest that you combine the instructors' teaching and personal experience, and your own inner sense of self in order to make the changes you desire.

2. *If you don't have good posture, what do you have?* How does your body feel to you? How would you describe your body? Your posture? Try it! Imagine you're describing someone else; be as objective as you can and draw in words how you think the world views your body/posture. After reading your description of the above posture, what do you think is the condition of its owner?

3. *Why do you think you carry your body in this way?* Although this question is harder, try not to skip over it. Think about it and write down your answer—it could be a very important tool in your learning process. Since our bodies reflect our opinions and conceptions about life, your posture could be giving you a clue on an attitude that needs attending to. As you're considering making some changes in your posture, you might want to include a change in the attitudes that have helped hold that posture.

4. *Why change what you already have?* Now that you've verbalized what you have, let's examine why you're willing to exert energy and time to change it. Are your reasons strictly cosmetic or are you actually physically uncomfortable? Is it your reflection in the store window that bothers you as you catch your image and think, "God, is that me?" When you put on your suit jacket, are your ears resting on your shoulders? When

you button your slacks or skirt, does your rib cage rest on your hips, hiding your waistline somewhere in between? Do your legs and feet get tired very easily? Does your lower back hurt? Do your shoulders and neck feel tense? Does the range of rotation of your head get smaller and smaller? Has someone told you all your life to sit up straight?

5. *Which parts of your body do you feel most in touch with?*

6. *Which parts do you like best? Why?*

7. *Which parts bother you?*

8. *Do you feel your body is an integrated part of yourself?*

9. *When you think of yourself, which parts of your body seem to represent your personality most?*

10. *What changes would you like to see happen?*

If your answer to this last question involves unrealistic wishing, examine your reasons for wishing this way. Sometimes setting impossible goals for yourself will only bring frustration and eventually end in defeat. A deterrent to self-improvement is an attitude of "hating your body." I can remember feeling "dissatisfied" with mine, which prompted me to learn about it and my concepts about it. This in turn taught me that I could have a voice in molding it and changing it. In my experience, people who are stuck in a "hate thing" with their bodies block off an important area of acceptance that then allows change to take place.

Realistic goals you've set for yourself can be achieved. Good posture is the result of a combination of self-knowledge, self-discipline, and self-confidence.

Chapter II

Self-awareness

Although this section is titled "Self-awareness," I have actually been dealing with self-awareness from the onset of this manual. The aspect of it I've dealt with so far has been in the intangible areas of thought and feelings that underlie posture and govern it. Let's move on to more tangible elements of self-awareness—pain and pleasure —which is how our thoughts and feelings manifest themselves in our physical awareness.

PHYSICAL AWARENESS

If the body is feeling good and functioning well, we are usually unaware of its existence. It serves us well, does our bidding, freeing our thoughts to deal with other areas of living. When we have a headache, we become painfully aware of our head. Likewise, if we become aware of our shoulders, neck, or lower back, we are getting a signal that something is amiss and should be attended to. Our concentration is then dragged back to the aching part of our anatomy. This is a protective kind of body awareness that is essential for our well-being. However, with a keener understanding of our body's signals, it is likely that we won't have to wait until there's pain to

16

realize that something is wrong. A daily awareness will build up our sensitivity to the signs along the way.

Another kind of body awareness that is also essential for our well-being comes not from pain but from pleasure and satisfaction. As your body responds to the exercises and you gain more awareness of your body, you will be on your way to a new self-confidence—a physical self-confidence that will allow you the joy, when undertaking a new physical activity, of knowing your body can handle and carry out your instructions. Everyone is entitled to these joyful experiences. All it takes is wanting it enough and working for it consistently.

In order to train yourself to understand your body's language and to appreciate its accomplishments, you must have patience. Realize that in undertaking this endeavor, you will need concentration and attention, and may have to hold off on other projects for a space of time. At the beginning you may feel as if all this concentration on your body is getting out of hand and you're becoming narcissistic. Don't worry, though; it just seems extreme compared to the kind of attention you gave this matter previously. As your new insights become incorporated into your life, your conscious efforts will be needed less and less.

THE PHYSICAL BODY

The mechanics of the body are complex and it would take years of study to begin to understand its workings. Fortunately, our learning process doesn't require that much input for physical change.

There are many motives for movement. As babies, we learn by observation and imitation. These tools continue to play a major role in learning throughout our lives. However, as we become more sophisticated and learn to compete, the desire to succeed becomes another motivation. Entangled with this desire is the ability to make changes in ourselves in order to achieve our goals, and making changes involves thought and examination.

Movement, and control of movement, begins in the nervous system. Once movement is learned, it becomes ingrained and stored there. When a stored coordination is required, the action involved for its performance takes place below the thinking level. To relearn or change the ingrained, stored movement is more complex. It's tricky to short-circuit or bypass the action that is below the thinking level. What gives us an edge is that our thoughts and feelings also originate in the nervous system. Through thought and images, we bring our imaginations into play to help us accomplish the bypass. Images conceived in our imagination have a quality of "pretending" that somehow touches the child in us and seemingly, magically, frees us to experience new things in the body.

It's like entering through another door, or digging a new pattern groove in the nervous system. In other words, we're tricking our computer, the nervous system! The images allow one to experience new skeletal placement and the exercises strengthen and lengthen the muscles which will stabilize the bones. A helpful image to use in improving our posture is to think in terms of our skeletons.

The answers you give to the following questions will give you an idea what your present concepts are in regard to your skeleton. Be as specific as you can in answering these questions.

The drawings and explanations that follow the questions will give you a modest framework about a very difficult and technical subject: how your body is put together and operates.

More Questions for Your Body Notebook:

1. *From what part of your body do you think your arms originate and move?*
2. *Where do you think your spine starts and ends?*
3. *What's the difference between your scapula and your shoulder?*
4. *From what part of your body do you think your legs originate and rotate?*
5. *Do you have the same awareness of your back as you do of the front of your body?*
6. *What is your contact to the ground? How well do you treat this part of your body, or even know it?*

The Skeleton
SKULL

As this manual appeals to your thought process, I thought it only fitting to introduce first the part of us where all thought originates.

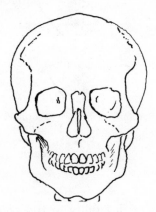

SPINE

Our spine is our upright carrier. It also houses and protects part of our nervous system. In the adult it is comprised of twenty-six separate bones called the vertebral column. The top seven are referred to as the cervical vertebrae and are generally known as the neck. The next twelve bones make up the thoracic vertebrae. The lower back or small of the back (lumbar region) contains five vertebrae. The sacrum, which is made up of five fused vertebrae and therefore considered one bone, is also the back part of the pelvic girdle. Last in line is the coccyx, four or five fused vertebrae also considered a single bone.

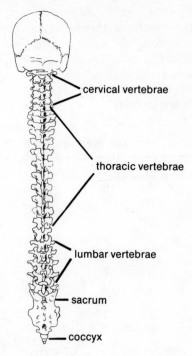

The amount of flexibility in the spine can readily be observed in children. The way the vertebrae articulate with each other allows forward, backward, and sideways movement. They are held securely together by ligaments. As the years go by and "play" gets lower on our list of priorities and our responsibilities take up more of our time, the spinal column gets little opportunity to exercise its full range of movement. The muscles supporting the spine get tighter not only from life's tensions but from lack of use. Gravity as well as daily tension contributes to our rounded shoulders. During the day, as we're standing upright, gravity compresses our spinal column, and by the end of the day, we are shorter than when we awoke in the morning. At night, lying flat, not having to resist gravity, the vertebrae are relieved of the pressure and decompress, making us taller in the morning.

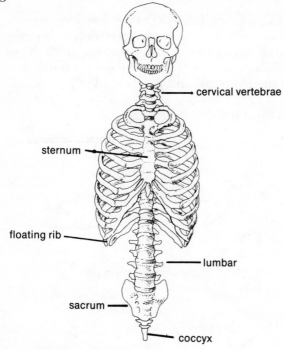

RIB CAGE

The rib cage is formed by twelve curved ribs attached in the back via cartilage and ligaments to the twelve thoracic vertebrae. In front, the top seven ribs are directly attached via cartilage to the sternum. The next three ribs are indirectly attached (via cartilage to the rib above), and then attached to the sternum. The eleventh and twelfth ribs are not attached at all to the sternum and are called floating ribs. The space the rib cage encircles is called the chest or thoracic cavity. It houses and protect numerous internal organs of the body. To get the feeling of a relaxed rib cage, a good visual image to use is to see the rib cage hanging from the spinal column. Aesthetically speaking, the rib cage is a lovely base on which to view a well-defined muscle structure.

CLAVICLE, SCAPULA, AND HUMERUS

A part of the body that seems generally vulnerable to tension and discomfort is the shoulder girdle. It comprises the clavicle, which joins the sternum in the front center of the rib cage, and the acromion process of the scapula. (When palpating your shoulder girdle it will be felt as the tip of the shoulder.) The scapulae are attached

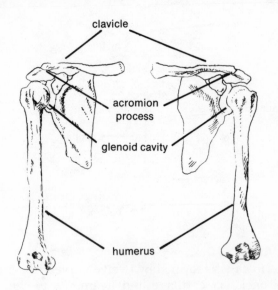

to the ribs in the back via muscles and tendons. The humerus (upper arm bone) articulates with the glenoid cavity of the scapula. Together they form a ball-and-socket type of joint. However, what is considered "just the shoulder" can't readily be seen on a skeleton as the shoulder is created by the various muscles and their wrappings covering the spaces created by parts of these bones.

SPINE, SKULL, RIB CAGE, AND ARMS

Even though technically some muscles that lift and move the upper arm are located in "the shoulder," there are more located in the scapula area. From this sketch, notice how inefficient the arms are without the clavicle and scapula. The most important point here is to make

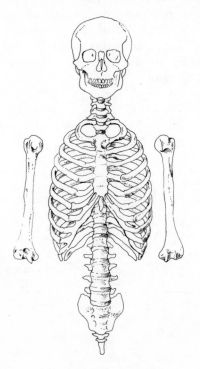

the connection in your thoughts that your arms originate with the scapula. One image to use while working on the shoulder girdle exercises is to see your arms growing out of your back like the wings of a bird.

PELVIC GIRDLE

In early life the hip bone (innominate bone) is made up of three separate bones: the ilium, the ischium and the pubis. Later, in the adult, the pelvic girdle is formed by the joining of the two hip bones. By means of strong ligaments, they join with the sacrum of the spinal column in the back, and in the front the two pubis bones join, also by cartilage. The joint of the two pubis bones is called symphysis pubis. However, in the exercises I use the term pubic bone instead of symphysis pubis. The space created below the rib cage and within the pelvic girdle is divided into two cavities: the abdominal cavity and the pelvic cavity. Within these cavities lie organs and intestines. Separating the thoracic cavity from the abdominal cavity is the important breathing muscle called the diaphragm.

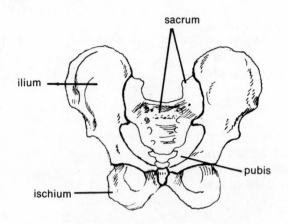

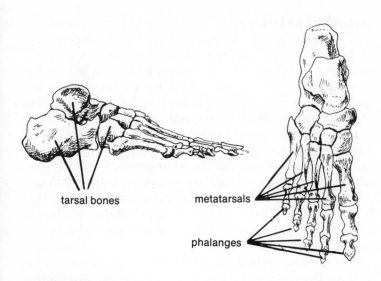

tarsal bones   metatarsals

phalanges

THE FOOT

Being our direct contact with the earth, our feet are
the base for carrying our weight. For doing this, we
should treat them more kindly than we do. Unfortunately, style dictates that looks are more important than
comfort and health; toes are crammed into odd shapes
that have more to do with the shoe designers' egos than
with our feet. Without exception, the people who work
in our studio need to reawaken the muscles in their feet.

In the front half of the foot there are five metatarsal
bones and fourteen phalanges. In the back half there are
seven larger bones called tarsal bones. It is the arch, and
the architectural construction of these bones, that allows
the foot, even though it is such a small part of us, to have
the large responsibility of carrying our weight. There are
longitudinal arches and transverse arches. While doing
the exercises, keep in mind that the best weight-bearing
position for the foot is the tripod of the foot. This triangle
is composed of the first metatarsal bone under the big
toe, the fifth metatarsal bone under the little toe and the
middle of the heel. Consciously be aware of its contact
with the floor.

THE SKELETON

After reading the skeletal description, it is important for you to study your body naked with your hands and your eyes. As the hands are our prime source of tactility, they will be helpful in giving you information. Make believe you're under the shower and have soapy hands and are washing yourself. Place your attention on feeling as much of your skeletal system as you can. Start with your head, behind your ears, down your neck, along your clavicle (collarbone), and down your sternum. Feel your ribs; try to find your floating ribs. Trace your pelvic girdle. Differentiate between your sacrum and your lumbar vertebrae. Try to find your coccyx. Differentiate between the cervical and the thoracic vertebrae; trace your scapula, humerus, and so on.

Then, examine your posture from many angles in the mirror. Try to observe yourself skeletally in the mirror. Mentally strip away your skin, muscles, veins, nerves, and organs. In your body notebook, try drawing your own skeleton.

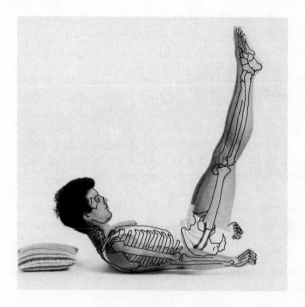

Breathing

At birth we begin breathing in a natural, rhythmic pattern called diaphragmatic breathing. Our psychological framework is formed by our early life experiences and these experiences dictate our behavior in later life. These same early life experiences structure our physicality, including how we carry ourselves and the ease or difficulty with which we breathe. From the moment we hold our breath with our first experience of anger, fear, or frustration, we set up the probability of a breathing pattern. As breathing is not something we dwell on or even check in the growing child (unless there are obvious problems), we arrive in adulthood with our breathing patterns set—whether or not they are uncomfortable or counterproductive.

When we're in a learning process, such as learning a new physical coordination, it is possible to experience fear, anger, and/or frustration. Often in this situation people will ask, "How should I be breathing?" What does this imply? Some need or fear in us is so strong that it blocks off what should be a natural, ongoing process of life—breathing. Whether we feel we need to be "great" at this new activity or feel nervous about being judged by others or ourselves as we learn it, we become anxious and find ourselves holding our breath.

I can't stress strongly enough how important it is to get a clear understanding of how you, individually, use this source of life. Unfortunately, the speed of and the demands of life do not encourage us to examine and explore what we think of as naturally ours. Yet, we could use our breath more to our advantage if we understood it! Become conscious of your breath and your breathing patterns as part of your self-observation.

Breathing Questions for Your Body Notebook:

1. *When you're lying in bed reading and relaxing, how would you describe your breathing? Be as specific as you can.*

2. *Compare the above description with how you breathe when you're afraid or frustrated.*
3. *How do you breathe when you are involved in a sport or any other competitive situation?*

For the reasons mentioned above and because of our incomplete communication with our inner sense of what's right, I feel there is confusion about breathing in general and about which breathing is best for which activity. Unless a person is directly involved with an activity connected with his or her breathing such as singing, playing a wind instrument, swimming, or yoga, he or she doesn't really have a point of reference from which to speak about breath. More often than not, people breathe shallowly (high chest breathing), which means they use the upper front part of their lungs only. However, when inhaling comfortably in diaphragmatic breathing, the diaphragm (which is a muscle) lowers and the rib cage expands laterally, allowing the lungs to fill with air. On exhalation the diaphragm and rib cage contract, helping the lungs expel the air. Naturally, there can be some movement in the abdominal wall and chest.

Science has been telling us for years that the average person does not use his or her full lung capacity. Yoga has been dealing with the breathing process for centuries, and serious students of Hatha Yoga study the importance of breathing while exercising. They practice various techniques to experience as much of their breathing capacity and potential as possible. They explore not only shallow breathing, but panting, single-lung isolation, back breathing, and deep abdominal breathing (D.A.B.). D.A.B. has gained much popularity, and is now being used in other forms of exercise. D.A.B. goes further than the diaphragmatic breathing. In D.A.B., the image used is to fill the lungs from the bottom up, which makes the abdominal wall extend a great deal. While resting I find this a very filling and satisfying sensation.

Unfortunately, the American way of life tends toward fads and quick, easy ways to achieve, so that valuable processes such as yoga are watered down for general consumption and inaccuracies and misconceptions take the place of knowledge. I believe that this happened in the case of D.A.B. Please note that I am not saying it's wrong to adapt what is appropriate for yourself from various philosophies and disciplines. In fact, I encourage this. What I urge is that you research well in order to have a clear understanding of what and why you're doing what you're doing. For example, if, while playing racquetball, you were to take a deep abdominal breath in anticipation of twisting to swing at the ball with your racket, excess stress would be placed on the lower back because your abdomen is distended with air. If the breath were taken more laterally and the abdominal wall was tautly supporting your innards, not only would your swing be stronger, but your day would be more pleasant because you would have no lower backache.

A basic requirement for continuing good posture is a strong abdominal wall to save unnecessary pressure and stress on the small of the back (lumbar region). What I'm suggesting for use in these posture exercises is a combination of basic diaphragmatic breathing and yoga back breathing. Imagine when inhaling that the air enters your nostrils and rides down the back of your neck. While it fills (extends) your sides, the front part of your body is comparatively unmoved. This will prove more difficult for some people than for others. I did not find it easy to master, but can assure you now that it has been well worth the time and effort. It required much concentration while doing the exercises, and more concentration while trying to involve it in the rest of my life. The hints and tricks in the Self-discipline section are what helped me finally to master it.

Chapter III

Self-discipline

What lies between wanting good posture and having good posture is obviously more complex than the connective word "and." It's self-knowledge, self-awareness, self-discipline and self-confidence.

We've all at one time or another, repeatedly, determined to make changes in our lives and after a week, or a month, reverted to our old habits. We pathetically put ourselves down for not having the will power to fulfill the change. What has to be decided first is *How much do I really want the change*? Do I want it only if it's easy? If I don't have to tax my brain, or possibly, my body? If someone else will do it for me or lead me?

We're capable of many things, and one of the more positive things is that we can initiate change. No longer is it excusable to hide behind "that's how I was born." Changing patterns in our life is not easy. It is more than just talking about it to our friends, convincing them and ourselves how earnest we are. After this paragraph, stop reading for a moment, and just sense what you are feeling—that inner knowing voice. All it requires to be heard or felt is space, quiet, time and attention. Maybe what you feel is that you want the change but feel too pressured in your life right now to instigate it. That's O.K., don't push; the book will be here when you're ready. If your inner voice says you are ready for the change, then read on.

HINTS AND TRICKS FOR PROCESSING CHANGE

Notes and Reminders

When I first decided to keep a body notebook, I soon realized that good intentions simply weren't enough for me. I'd start out the day with my body notebook in my pocketbook, determined to jot down some reactions at least once during the day. I'd unpack in the evening at home, when, lo and behold, I'd take out this strange book and think, "What the hell is this?" After a few days of this, I came up with the idea of making notes to myself on small index cards or scraps of paper. I'd use brightly colored inks and catchy, funny, or even serious quotes and reminders which I would put in strategic places to attract my attention. I had these notes on my bathroom mirror, my refrigerator, in my change purse, taped in my briefcase, taped inside my desk drawer, on my pocket mirror, taped inside my hat or wrapped inside my lunch. Instead of the label at the neck of my coat, I'd see a message to think of my scapula until I got home! It became a source of relaxation and self-amusement to come up with clever comments that were going to help me. From the notes and reminders I had no trouble remembering to use the body notebook.

"Notes and Reminders" grew into a more elaborate and sophisticated process as I worked on individual parts of my body. I would choose one part on which I was concentrating and decide for that day it would be my focus. Prepared for this, I would have my notes and reminders written and ready and knew that in any spare fleeting moment I would shift my concentration to that particular part and see if I were doing what I was supposed to be doing with it (i.e., relaxing my shoulder). I remember hysterical moments at the onset of this program when I would panic, thinking there was something very important that I was forgetting, and then laugh

with relief when I realized it was just my posture proj-
ect! I was so delighted that I hadn't messed up somewhere that it even became more of a pleasure to
incorporate my posture chore for the day!

Layering

Layering is the adding on of one thought over another.
When learning a new physical coordination, people are
often surprised to find it more difficult to perform than
they thought. Because of their own lack of forethought
about what is involved in the movement, people get frustrated, lose interest, and give up. Layering is a way to
deal with these frustrations and allows the person to
learn how to learn.

In order to "layer on," you must first break down the
whole exercise into its parts. As it's impossible to disen-
gage one working part of the body from another, what
we're actually disengaging is our attention from the
whole to one of its parts.

EXAMPLE: In working on a spine awareness exercise
(see Chapter IV, "The Exercises"), I will ask you to keep
your attention on your spine—to sense its flexibility, its
tightness, its curves, its straightness, and so on. In pur-
suing this line of thought, out the window goes your
abdominal awareness and your breathing awareness.

It's okay! Keep your focus where you want it and just
get familiar with your spine. Don't make judgments or
have recriminations because you can't do two things at
once. You'll learn. That's what this book is about. After
a while, with this kind of repetition, you'll be able to
sense your spine from a peripheral point of your attention and be ready to put the center of your attention on
another part of the whole (i.e., abdomen or breathing).
And after another while you will even be able to shift
your attention from one to the other and make any nec-
essary corrections.

Mental Tapes

A mental tape is like a cassette tape loop which runs in your mind. Making a mental tape was my way of dealing with the barrage of thoughts that kept interfering with my concentration and ultimately held me back from accomplishing what I wanted. It is the setting of your thought process to repeat over and over again a prewritten script of limited instructions that will block out other thoughts while you are doing an exercise. In order to arrive at the most helpful script of instructions for your situation, it is important not only to understand the exercise, but also to understand your body's needs.

An example of assessing a postural situation and writing a mental tape for an exercise is illustrated on page 37, in the section called "Planning Your Own Program."

Mental Tapes/Layering—Out in the World

This is a game I'd play while en route—anywhere. I'd choose a specific change I wanted to make—for example, to keep my shoulders from curling forward toward my chest. I'd prepare an image that gave me the best sense of placement. Example: A stream of heavy water rushing out of my ears, traveling the length of my shoulders, tumbling down my upper arms. This image was enough to enable me to keep my shoulders feeling more comfortably placed. I then had to deal with doing this in the street and not looking like a sleepwalker. This was tricky, for I find when I'm concentrating hard on something I get a faraway look in my eyes. So I'd use the mental tape concept. I interspersed my awareness of walking in the street with my mental image, then I would switch back to walking in the street, then back to the image, and so on. Repeating this a few days in a row made it much easier to practice while walking. I was gradually able to continue the process through the trip to work. (It took a long time to incorporate this action while at work!)

Standing in a bus or subway, holding onto a handle overhead, was a good place to examine what was happening in my shoulder girdle while my arms were over my head. I didn't want my shoulders up around my ears, so I used the image of lifting my arms out of my back (like a bird lifts its wings) to relax my shoulder.

While waiting for an elevator and then riding in it, I'd practice lateral back breathing while using my abdominal wall as a support for my lower back. Each time I did these things I increased the length of time I was able to incorporate the changes into my everyday life.

CHAPTER IV

The Exercises

We've examined the feelings and attitudes you have about your body. We've talked about the nervous system, skeletal system, breathing concepts, and we have learned how to include observational discipline in your daily lives. Now let's take a look at your thoughts about exercise—the calorie-burning, energy exerting, physical output which is unavoidable if change is to actually happen.

According to the dictionary, exercise is:

1. A setting in action or practicing: use; habitual activity, occupation
2. Exertion for the sake of training or improvement, whether physical, intellectual or moral; specifically bodily exertion for keeping the organs and functions healthy
3. To exert or practice for the sake of training or improvement as the wits or limbs; to subject to discipline, to put in practice

COMMON MISCONCEPTIONS REGARDING EXERCISE

Throughout my years of teaching exercises, I've met a variety of people who've had misconceptions regarding

35

exercise. The following list (with the exception of number 6) includes types of people whose attitudes are the ones I've found to be negative, the people who hadn't a chance to succeed from the minute they walked in, unless they would begin to recognize how their attitudes were standing in the way of their progress.

1. The people who sign up for a class and think it's their responsibility to get their bodies there, change from their business clothes into the appropriate gym garment, and then put their bodies into the hands of the instructor. Meanwhile, their thinking process goes out to lunch.

2. Overly self-concerned people who have trouble accepting the natural aging process are others who are doing themselves harm. They feel that they'll never be what they were ten years ago. Of course, they won't, they're going to be something else and it doesn't necessarily have to be less. They get caught in a web of their fears and tensions, however, and just what they fear, they perpetuate.

3. We all know people who are just consumers at heart. They love buying gadgets and outfits, but their interest wanes as soon as the buying spree is over and the nitty-gritty begins.

4. There are people who feel the more strenuous the activity, the more violently they twist, turn, squirm, sweat, jerk, but above all keep moving hard, the more they are exercising!

5. Then there is the category of people who exercise under extreme pressure of guilt. After forty minutes, the guilt lifts and they don't find the drive to exercise for another two weeks (until the proper amount of guilt has built up).

6. Most people, however, are simply ignorant about how their bodies are put together and how they work. With the desire to improve and learn about themselves, this group of people are the easiest to change.

PLANNING YOUR OWN PROGRAM

Now that I've encouraged you to keep a body diary, I'll discuss how it can help you design your own program. First of all, *Don't stop writing in it!* Whether you realize it or not, through observing yourself and recording your findings, you have been laying the groundwork for your posture program. Read the notebook through many times with a careful eye and not a self-deprecating one. You may have found it helpful to have been the self-watcher for anywhere from a week to two months. This is an important aspect of the plan. If you make just a token gesture of observing, you won't have enough information from which to evaluate and work. It's okay, too, to spend anywhere from a few days to a few weeks, or even months, just working with your breathing. Then, when ready, move on. After reading this book completely and getting an idea of the progression of the objectives of the book, lay out a "temporary" program for yourself. (Of course, before beginning any exercise program it is wise to check with your doctor.)

1. Your first decision should be how often you intend to exercise and for how long. The minimum would be twice weekly and optimum would be four times. There's nothing wrong with every day, but don't set yourself up for not achieving by setting unrealistic goals.

2. How long will each session be? What will your schedule allow, and how much can your concentration handle? Anywhere from fifteen to thirty minutes is fine. Write it in your schedule for the week in big letters—EXERCISE! Give it its place and time so you can't dismiss it easily.

3. Where will you be exercising? Choose a place where you feel physically comfortable and separate from your family or roommates, so you'll be able to concentrate seriously on yourself.

4. What you'll need: A full-length mirror would be

helpful, an exercise pad or substitute, such as a folded blanket or towels (so you are comfortable while rolling on your spine), a straightback chair close by, a small hard pillow, and a towel.

5. The ideal progression of your daily session: On pages 40–41 you'll find a list of exercises. Start with the first exercise in each section. Add the next exercise in each section as you feel you are satisfied with your understanding and performance of the previous one. It's okay if you progress faster in some sections than you do in others.

6. Read through the exercises you will be working on a few times. Try them out. Observe while doing them which areas of your body need the most attention. Make a list of these areas. Now you're going to write a mental tape to assist you in working on those areas. Following is a description of an exercise and two examples of mental tapes. Each involve a different area, but both involve breathing. After getting one area under control you can use the second example to deal with the next confused area.

PELVIC TILT

Original position: Sit on mat, knees bent, feet parallel and in line with hips, standing consciously on the tripod of the foot. Heels are eighteen to twenty-four inches from buttocks. Back is straight. Arms are held out in front of you, shoulder width, high and wide, palms down.

Action: Lower vertebrae, one at a time. Coccyx is down, next comes sacrum and then lumbar. Reverse action: Lumbar comes off mat, then the sacrum and end by sitting tall in original position.

Objective: Stretch lower spine, thereby strengthening abdominal muscles, breathing comfortably and not involving the shoulder girdle during the action of exercise.

Notes and Comments: Think of tilting pubic bone to chin while lowering vertebrae to mat. Make up an image for yourself, something like: The only way your abdominal muscles can help you will be if they are falling into the cavity of your pelvis and pressing the spine down.

If part of my assessment of my posture was that (1) I had a tight lower back, (2) held tension in my shoulders, and (3) also tended to hold my breath, I would have chosen to concentrate on my breathing and shoulders first. The italicized words make up my mental tape. The words in parentheses are not part of the mental tape, but just a description of where, within the action of the exercise, I would use the mental tape.

a. *Inhale* (in my back and sides)
   Check shoulders (before action begins)
b. *Exhale* (lowering one vertebra at a time)
   Check shoulders
c. *Inhale* (while still down)
   Check shoulders
d. *Follow exhale up* (to original position)
   Check shoulders

Now I will rewrite the tape to concentrate on the tightness in the lower back. Again, the words in parentheses are not the mental tape, but instructions for when to incorporate the mental tape.

a. (before action of exercise begins)
   Inhale (in back and sides)
   Abdomen pressing against spine

b. (stretching out lower back)
   Exhale (tip pubic bone toward chin)
   Abdominal muscles pressing vertebrae to mat

c.   (while still down)
   Inhale
   Abdomen pressing spine
      down
d. *Exhale brings you up*   (to original position)
   Abdominal muscles
      glued to spine

You can adapt and personalize each exercise for your needs by writing your own mental tapes. In the description of the exercises, I have stated what the exercise is designed to achieve, but even within this frame of reference, the emphasis will be different. Each person doing the exercise will use a variation of the directions, as a result of his or her particularly diagnosed needs. Using your own mental tape will help you "layer" new physical coordination into the part of your nervous system where the change must be registered. This approach of breaking things down and dealing with one thing at a time leads to the layers becoming a part of you. You will get a clearer sense of what is actually happening in your body during the exercise.

After you've done the exercises for a month or two, start incorporating what you're sensing and learning into your daily life other than just when you are exercising. Use the Notes and Reminders described in Chapter III, or better yet, ideas you have come up with during this learning period. This way the exercise program is strictly yours and comes from your own center of self.

THE EXERCISES

I. Breathing
   1. Basic Back Breathing
   2. Basic Lateral Breathing 1
      Basic Lateral Breathing 2

Basic Lateral Breathing 3
Basic Lateral Breathing 4
Basic Lateral Breathing 5
3. Breathing Spine
II. Hands
1. Fingers
2. Palm Stretch
3. Samson Exercise
4. Fingers—Scapula Connection

III. Neck Awareness
1. Weighted Forehead
2. Weighted Ear
3. Neck Twist

IV. Feet Awareness
1. Toe Separation
2. Metartarsal Drag
3. Towel Drag

V. Shoulder Girdle Awareness
1. Shoulder Roll
2. Half-Scapula Lift
3. Scapulae Lift
4. Rooster Stretch
5. Forearm-Scapula
6. Backward Arm Pull
7. Towel Stretch

VI. Spine Awareness
1. Hand Hold
2. Spine Pull
3. Spine Reach
4. Pelvic Tilt
5. Pelvic Lift and Lower
6. Rolling Through the Spine
7. Back Straights

I. Breathing

NOTES ON THE BREATHING EXERCISES

The position for the first breathing exercise is to allow you to experience filling your back and sides easily. Exercises Basic Lateral Breathing 1–5 are one exercise broken down into workable segments, layering one body awareness upon another. First read through them all so you'll understand the objective, then practice BBB. Add BLB 1. Try to get some sensation in your back and sides while in this position. Begin each exercising session with the BBB until you feel you don't need it to set you up for BLB 1. When you can start with BLB 1 and feel confident with your breath in the back and sides, progress to BLB 2. If you lose the sensation, try BBB to get it back again and proceed.

The last breathing exercise is quite complex. Please don't play with it until you are satisfied with your understanding of BLB 5 and have started Spine Awareness exercises. This exercise not only involves practicing breathing in different areas of the body via the spine but uses the breath to allow the muscles to stretch without forcing or pushing. It's meditative in nature and can take anywhere from fifteen to thirty minutes by itself.

Sometimes in breathing exercises some people experience hyperventilation. This is an excess of oxygen reaching the blood and an abnormal loss of carbon dioxide leaving the blood. The symptoms are dizziness and light-headedness. If you feel hyperventilated, simply rest for a minute or two until it passes and then continue. This should stop as you move along in your program.

1. BASIC BACK BREATHING

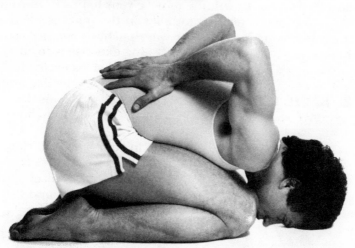

Original Position: Sit with your knees bent and legs under you, forehead resting on the mat. Place the heels of your hands on your lower ribs with your fingers pointing toward your backside. Close your eyes.

Action: When you breathe, imagine your breath taking the following course: Inhale through your nose; breath travels behind your ears, down the back of your neck, and fills your back and not your front. Inhale to the count of five (count silently), and exhale to the count of five. (Remember, you're inhaling through your nose and exhaling through your mouth, but feel free to exhale through your nose if it feels more comfortable.) Your goal is to take ten complete breaths. However, it is all right to start with however many you can handle correctly and work your way up to the full ten.

Objective: To experience the sensation when you fill your back and sides with air and leave your chest and abdomen comparatively uninvolved.

Notes and Comments: Being in this position will help you sense your back filling as you are folded over and compressing the front of you. When you feel somewhat secure with the breathing, remove your hands from your sides and rest them comfortably on the mat. Sense the breath in your back as if it were pushing against your hands.

2. BASIC LATERAL BREATHING 1

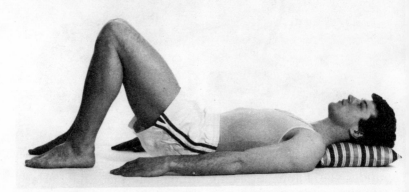

Original Position: Lie on your back with your head on a small pillow, knees bent, feet consciously making contact with the floor, and the small of your back (lumbar region) resting on mat.

Action: When you breathe, imagine the air entering your nose, traveling behind your ears, down the back of your neck, and filling the back of you and not the front of you. Do ten complete breaths.

Objective: Same as for BBB.

Notes and Comments: This exercise is a step more advanced than the previous one. In this exercise the position of the body will not help as much and you'll need more concentration. Now, let me just say again, *This is not easy,* so don't despair. Concentrate on what you are doing—it gets easier. To test yourself, place your hands on the sides of your rib cage (even with your chest). As you inhale, feel your ribs expand laterally and watch your abdominal wall staying as near to quiet as possible. You may become aware that you fill more naturally on one side than another. That's okay. Just consciously direct your breath to fill the other side. Then direct it to fill evenly. At the beginning, this could feel quite uncomfortable. Learning to coordinate something new into an already existing system of behavior isn't easy.

BASIC LATERAL BREATHING 2

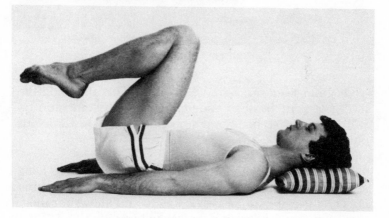

Original Position: Same as BLB 1, except knees are lifted toward the chest.

Objective: Concentrate on allowing the abdominal wall to sink to the spine and stay quiet as you proceed with the lateral breathing.

BASIC LATERAL BREATHING 3

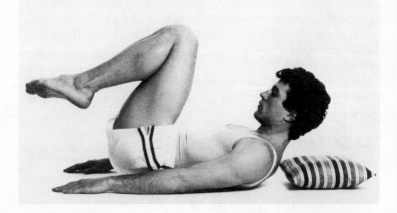

Original Position: Same as BLB 2. This time add the lifting of your head to your chest. Reach your chin toward your pubic bone and your pubic bone toward your chin.

Objective: Same as for BLB 2.

Notes and Comments: As your chin and pubic bone are reaching for each other, sense how this reaching deepens the abdomino-pelvic cavity and allows for more depth for your abdominal wall to fall into.

BASIC LATERAL BREATHING 4

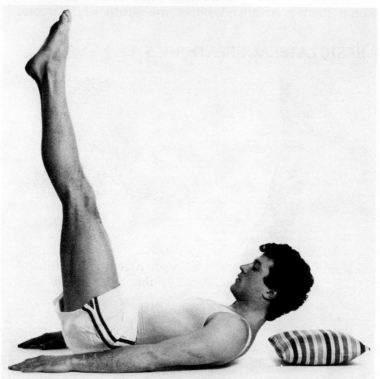

Original Position: Same as BLB 3, plus we're adding more abdominal work. Keeping your lower back resting on the mat, extend your straight legs upward, trying to keep the insides of your thighs touching, aiming your toes toward the point where the ceiling meets the wall.

Objective: Same as BLB 2.

Notes and Comments: DO NOT BITE OFF MORE THAN YOU CAN CHEW. If you feel your back coming away from the mat, change the angle of your legs (bringing them closer to your head) to insure that your lower back rests on the mat. It is more important that the back be resting on the mat than that your legs be held aloft.

If you are impatient and want to skip the basics and get on with more advanced things, your attitude is all wrong.

BASIC LATERAL BREATHING 5

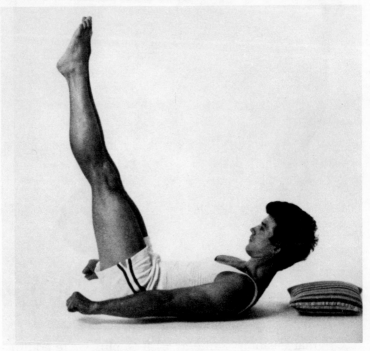

Original Position: Start with the same as BLB 4. The last addition to this exercise is the incorporation of the shoulder girdle. With straight arms and a closed fist, stretch your arms long out of the scapula. Slowly pump your arms up and down in rhythm with your breath. (The movement must originate from the scapula and not the neck muscles or forearms.)

Objective: Same as BLB 2.

3. BREATHING SPINE

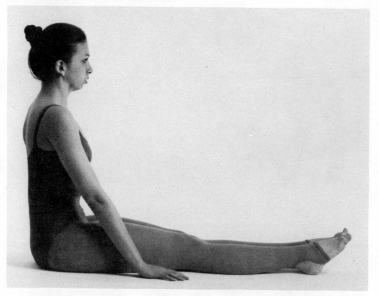

Original Position: Sit on carpet or exercise mat with legs straight out in front of you. Let hands rest on floor by sides of knees.

Objective: To experience the sensations involved while using the breath for stretching.

Notes and Comments: This is a slow-moving exercise and the stretch is achieved best with concentration on the breath. Imagine that your forehead is weighted and is being pulled down toward your knees. Start becoming aware of your breath. Mentally watch the breath enter your nose and ride down the back of your curved neck and spine. On the exhalation, feel the air being helped out as your ribs compress and the width of your back slackens. As your forehead lowers, slide your hands on the floor toward your calves. If this is not easy, just leave them where they are. Inhale again, feeling the air enter your nose, travel down the neck, fill the back down to the small of your back. As you exhale, again feel your

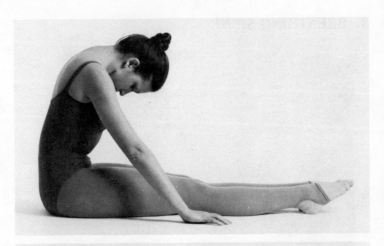

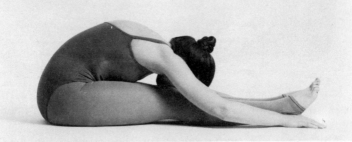

back narrowing and, if possible, your head dropping forward toward your knees. Continue inhaling and exhaling, consciously following the new breath coming and going through your body. Please do not push this exercise—don't be impatient. It took me three months of daily practice to be able to lie my forehead and upper torso flat on my legs without any strain. When you're feeling ready to stop this stretch, come out of it the same way you got into it: *Very Slowly*. Try reversing your breathing. Imagine you are breathing through your toes and the breath is traveling up your legs, around your buttocks, into your lower back, through your spine, and lifts you up to a sitting position.

II. Hands

1. FINGERS

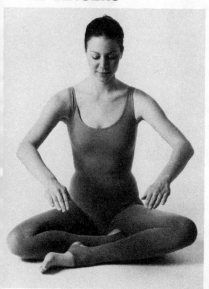 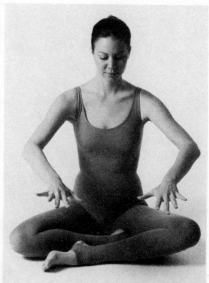

Original Position: Hold arms and hands outstretched in front of you, palms down to floor.

Action: (1) Stretch fingers out and apart and then pull together.

(2) Make believe you are playing an imaginary piano. Repeat several times, then palms up and repeat.

Objective: To become aware of and increase the flexibility in the fingers.

2. PALM STRETCH

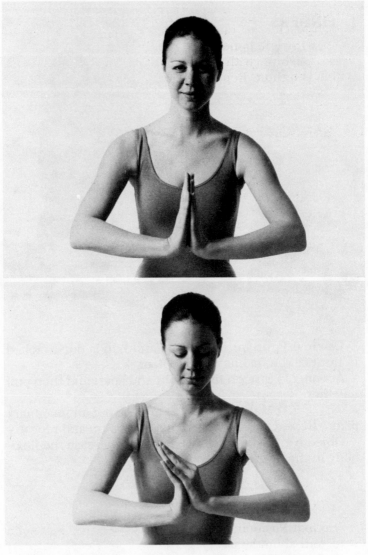

Original Position: Press palms and fingers together.
Action: Let right hand relax while left fingers press right fingers backward.

Objective: To stretch and strengthen finger and palm muscles.

Notes and Comments: Try not to involve shoulders, neck muscles, or elbows, but just isolate the fingers. Push with left hand and stretch with right. Then reverse, pushing with right and stretching left. Observe which is tighter. Repeat up to ten times on each side.

3. SAMSON EXERCISE

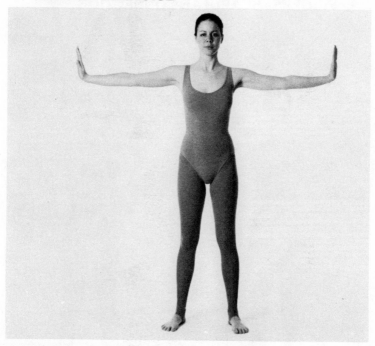

Original Position: Hold hands out to your side, even with your shoulders.

Action: Press your hands, from the heel of the palm to the straight tips of the fingers, solidly against imaginary walls.

Objective: To stretch the muscles in hand, wrist, and forearm.

Notes and Comments: Pretend you are Samson holding up the pillars of the temple. It will probably be a big stretch for you. Hold for the count of ten and then relax. Repeat five times.

4. FINGERS–SCAPULAE CONNECTION

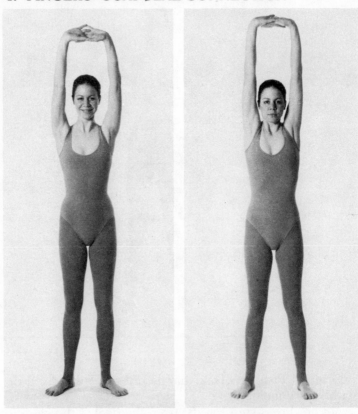

Original Position: Entwine your fingers, palms up to the ceiling, feet parallel, shoulder width apart.

Action: Reach with the palms to the ceiling to the point where your shoulders are involved and are up around your ears. Now focus on the scapulae and bring the shoulders down. Repeat.

Objective: To become aware of the connection from your scapulae to your fingers.

Notes and Comments: Don't pull your palms down from the top of the shoulders but bring them down with the scapulae.

III. Neck Awareness

1. WEIGHTED FOREHEAD

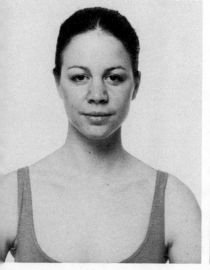
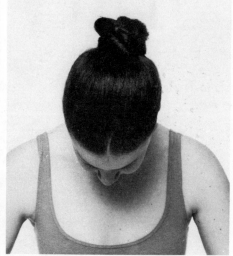

Original Position: Sit comfortably, Indian fashion, or with legs straddled over chair or stool. Arms resting comfortably.

Action: Imagine that your forehead is weighted and is slowly pulling your head forward toward your chest and stretching your neck (cervical area of spine). To return head to original position, imagine individual vertebrae are balls that will float one on top of the other. Repeat as often as you like!

Objective: To have the action feel as if you were not using your muscles at all, and to experience a lovely floating sensation.

Notes and Comments: At the beginning, do this in front of a mirror to make sure you are floating up straight.

2. WEIGHTED EAR

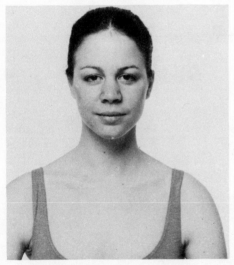 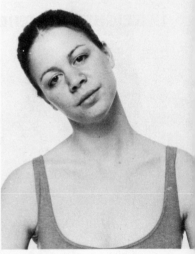

Original Position: Sit comfortably, Indian fashion, or with legs straddled over chair or stool. Arms resting comfortably.

Action: Think your left ear is weighted and it pulls the head toward the left shoulder. Nose acts as a pivot and right shoulder must not move to accommodate head falling to left. To return head to original position, imagine individual vertebrae are balls floating up, one on top of the other. Repeat five times on each side.

Objective: To strengthen and stretch neck muscles and release tension in this area.

3. NECK TWIST

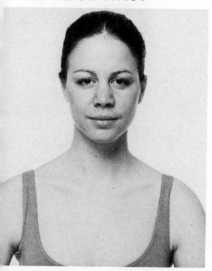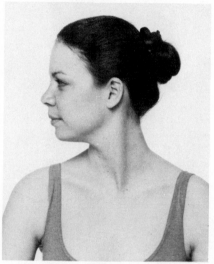

Original Position: Sit comfortably. Eyes straight ahead.

Action: Very slowly let eyes lead your head to the left, keeping shoulders facing forward. Go as far as you can without straining. Then let eyes bring you back to original position. This time let the image control be external . . . imagine what you're looking at is drawing your head around. Repeat five times. Then twist to the right five times.

Objective: Releasing tight grasp of neck muscles. Strengthening and stretching.

Notes and Comments: As you learn to use your arms from your scapulae and not from your shoulders and neck, this exercise will be more pleasant.

IV. Feet Awareness

1. TOE SEPARATION

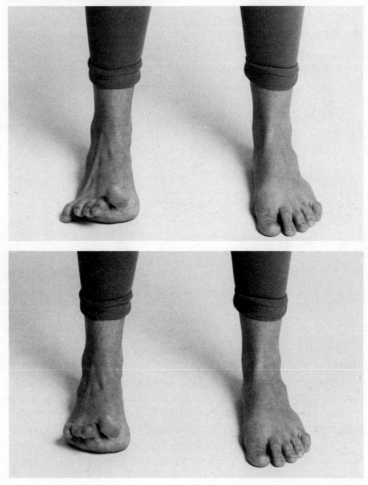

Original Position: Sit comfortably where you can handle your feet.

Action: Lift toes off floor keeping your heel and metatarsal bones on the floor. Slowly put one toe down at a time, beginning with the little toe, then the fourth, middle, second, big toe. Lift up one at a time starting with big toe, second, middle, fourth, little toe. Repeat five times. Repeat using other foot five times.

Objective: To use your toes as you do your fingers.

Notes and Comments: More often than not, the small toe does not respond. Use your hands to help awaken it. Pull it away from the other toes until you feel some sensation, then let it go. Now try to reproduce the sensation without using your hands. If nothing happens, do it again. Repeat until you see some life there. Even if it's just a nod, it's a beginning! I've never yet had a client who couldn't achieve this if they were willing to work at it.

2. METATARSAL DRAG

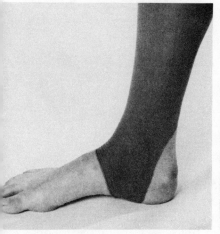 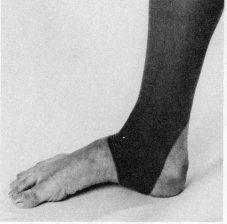

Original Position: If possible, do this on a floor that has lines in it, like wood or tile. Place the back of your heel perpendicular to a line. Again, sit comfortably so you can handle toes. During the action, the heel should not move over the line on the floor.

Action: Drag metatarsal to heel without crunching up toes or lifting metatarsal off the floor. The long arch of your foot will be lifted, but your metatarsal will not. Then, spread metatarsal bones and toes out as if you were standing on hot sand. Repeat five times on each foot.

Notes and Comments: If toes won't stay long but tend to curl up as you drag, lay fingers over them to help them stay long.

3. TOWEL DRAG

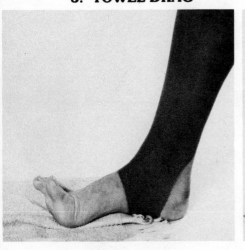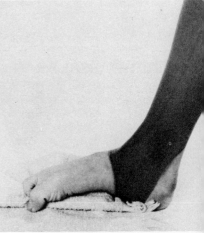

Original Position: Sit comfortably where you can handle toes. Lay towel on floor.

Action: Using what you learned from the previous exercises, lift toes, leaving heel and metatarsal bones down. Spread your toes and think of grabbing the towel (with the metatarsal arch) and pulling it toward you. Spread and lift toes to grab again. Don't be timid! Make it feel—you're using muscles that have been dormant for a while. They'll complain for a time, but then will get used to moving.

Notes and Comments: To make this more difficult (when the right time comes) place a weight—such as a heavy book—on the end of the towel and drag the towel with the added weight.

V. Shoulder Girdle Awareness

1. SHOULDER ROLL

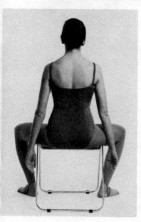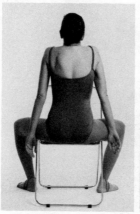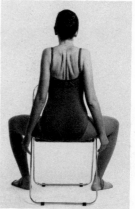

Original Positon: Sit Indian fashion or straddling a chair or stool, hands resting comfortably at your sides or on your knees.

Action: Let your shoulders roll forward into chest. Roll shoulders up to ears. Feel scapulae bring them down behind or in line with your ears. Repeat. Then reverse by rolling shoulders back first. Repeat five times each way.

Objective: Sensing the entire shoulder girdle and leaving rib cage at rest.

2. HALF-SCAPULA LIFT

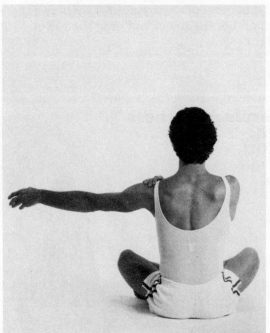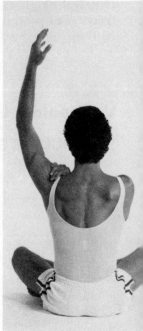

Original Position: Sit Indian fashion or straddling a chair or stool. Left arm is comfortably by your side. Place right hand cupped over left shoulder.

Action: Reaching out of your scapula, allow left arm to float up above your head. As the movement begins, palm faces forward, elbow is slightly bent and lifted to ceiling. At top of movement, palm is angled toward top of head. As you lower the arm, sense the work initiating in your scapula. Switch arms.

Objective: Keep left shoulder quiet in right cupped hand.

Notes and Comments: There will be some movement under your hand but basically your shoulder will not be rising up toward your ear to lift the arm. After you feel satisfied that you understand how to do the lift from the scapula in this half position, proceed to Scapulae Lift, using both arms together.

3. SCAPULAE LIFT

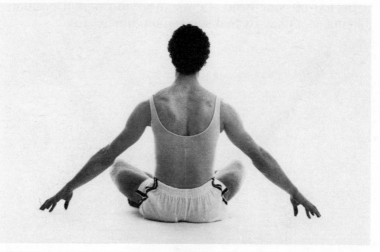

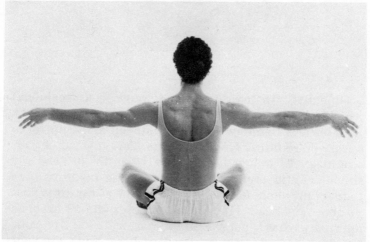

Original Position: Sit Indian fashion or straddling a chair or stool. Arms are comfortably by your side.

Action: During the movement, palms face forward, elbows are slightly bent and lifted to the ceiling (without rotating shoulders forward to lift elbows). Reaching out of your scapulae, your fingers meet above your head with arms fairly straight and the palms of your hands facing the top of your head. Lower arms to original position using scapulae. Repeat seven more times.

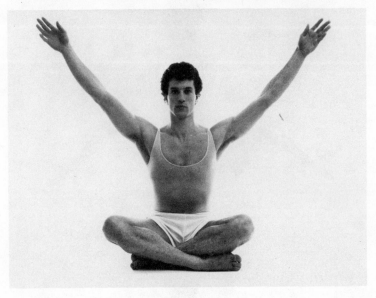

Objective: To use the area in your back (scapulae) which you sensed in the previous exercise.

Notes and Comments: Watch yourself in the mirror to see if you're lifting from your shoulders instead of your scapulae. An image I have found helpful to keep my shoulders still as my scapulae are lifting my arms is to think of my shoulders falling behind me as my arms float up above my head. Then I close my eyes and try to sense internally what I just saw in the mirror. If you find your shoulder area is close to head or ears, don't lift your hands any higher. Work within a range of correctness rather than completeness.

4. ROOSTER STRETCH

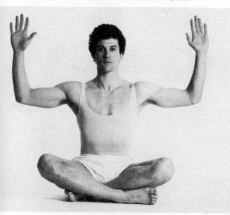 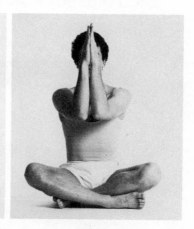

Original Position: Sit Indian fashion or straddling a chair or stool. Arms held out in an even line with your shoulders supported from scapulae. Arms are bent at elbows, hands pointing up with palms facing forward.

Action: Move arms forward toward each other, so that the forearms from inside elbow to tips of fingers touch. Elbows will be even with the middle of your chest. Draw them back to original position. Repeat.

Objective: To sense what is happening to your scapulae as your forearms meet in front of you. Your back is opening wide and your shoulders may feel a little forward. As your arms move back to the original position, allow your rib cage to stay relaxed.

Notes and Comments: Try to imagine how your scapulae look as you do this exercise.

5. FOREARM-SCAPULA

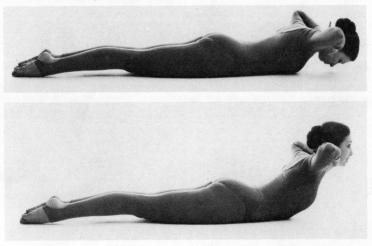

Original Position: Lie on your stomach with a small pillow under your abdomen to protect lower back from arching. Put fingers on side of neck, elbows pointing out to the side in back of or just in line with your ears.

Action: Lift your head and eyes while elbows wing back, thinking of keeping your neck long. Count to five, then roll down to original position. Repeat five times.

Objective: To strengthen the back and gain more sensitivity in the scapula area.

Notes and Comments: Still face down, put hands by shoulders and push yourself back, bending knees and sit on your heels, curving your back in the opposite direction for a release.

6. BACKWARD ARM PULL

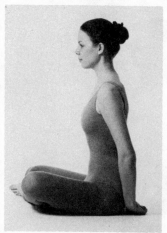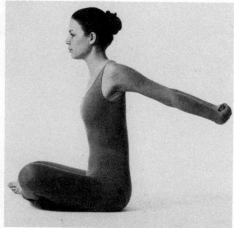

Original Position: Sit Indian fashion or straddling a chair or stool. Left hand is holding right hand resting on seat behind your back.

Action: Lift arms up (from their source, the scapula) and straight out behind you UNTIL you feel the need to change your shoulders and head position in order to accommodate arm lift. Hold lifted position for a count of five. Lower hands to original position. Repeat four more times. Switch hands and repeat action.

Objective: Lift arms up behind you, attempting to keep them straight with upper trunk in alignment. Don't let shoulders roll forward or rib cage stick out.

Notes and Comments: Do not make jerky movements. Put your concentration first on the sensations you're experiencing in the scapulae and then check your shoulders and rib cage.

7. TOWEL STRETCH

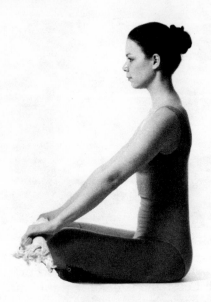

Original Position: Sit Indian fashion or straddling chair or stool. Hold rolled towel taut overhead with arms fairly straight (*Do not hyperextend elbows*), supported from scapulae and not from shoulders.

Action: Lower your arms behind you, keeping them as straight as you can. Then bring them forward in front of your head.

Objective: Feel the stretch in pectorals and upper arm and feel rotation originate from scapulae.

Notes and Comments: When you feel ready you can try the advanced version of this exercise. Stand up with knees slightly bent and back straight. Watch yourself in a mirror so you don't arch your back and stick out your rib cage as your arms go behind you. The closer together you hold your hands on the towel, the harder the exercise becomes. Please be careful. This is more difficult than it looks and if not approached intelligently, it can cause trouble.

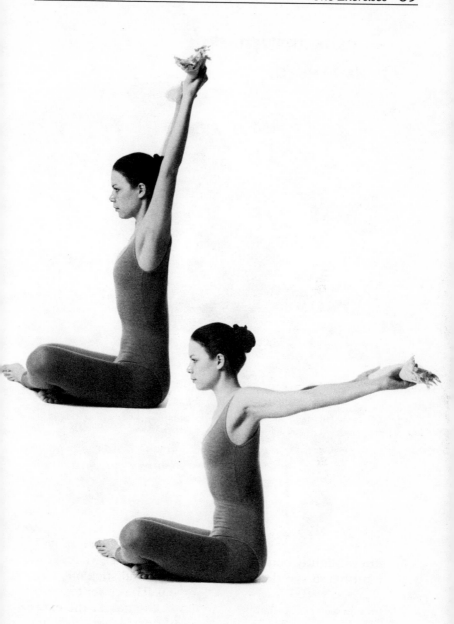

VI. Spine Awareness

1. HAND HOLD

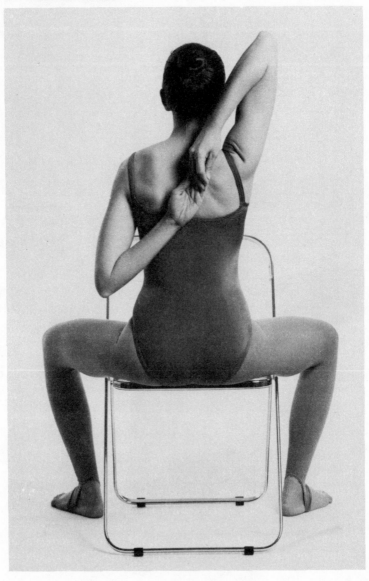

Original Position: Sit Indian fashion or straddling a chair or stool.

Action: Using your fingertips, feel around just below the middle of the back of your head. Find where your spine begins. With one hand, using fingertips gently, trace down your spine, being conscious of touching each vertebra. Your elbow ends pointing to the ceiling. With the other hand, move fingertips gently up your spine starting from its base until your fingers meet and try to hold hands. Now switch hands.

Objective: Holding hands behind your back, draw lower placed elbow back and upper elbow to ceiling, keeping rib cage in alignment. This is a very good stretch!

Notes and Comments: Chances are you will not be able to touch hands or you will be tighter on one side than the other. It's okay if you can't touch in the beginning. As you proceed, you will loosen up and stretch out.

2. SPINE PULL

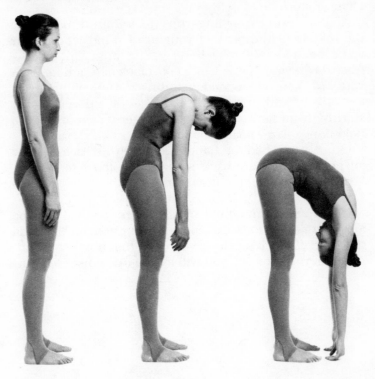

Original Position: Stand with feet shoulder width apart, arms hanging loosely by your sides.

Action: Imagine a weighted forehead as you did in the neck exercises. Let the weight just pull you down and forward gently, being aware of your vertebrae, one by one being pulled and stretched. When you've gone as far as is comfortable, and I do mean comfortable, start reversing the roll and come up . . . very slowly . . . vertebra by vertebra. If it hurts or pulls too much, you've gone too far. Your shoulders will drop into place because of the weight of your arms hanging by your side. Exhale on way down and inhale on way up.

Objective: To become conscious of the spine's rolling action.

3. SPINE REACH

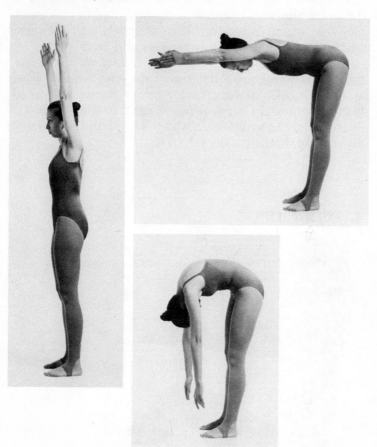

Original Position: Stand with feet shoulder width apart.

Action: Lift arms up to the ceiling, palms forward. *Don't lock knees.* Buttocks move backward as if being pulled, while you bend forward from your hips, consciously keeping your spine straight. After arriving at a ninety-degree angle, let the top of your body (leading with your arms) drop forward so your head and body are folded over your legs. *Don't lock knees.* Roll up as you did in the previous exercise. Arms will drop to your sides as you bring shoulders into alignment. Repeat five times.

Objective: More spine awareness and fluidity.

Notes and Comments: Reach for ceiling with your fingertips, keeping your abdominal muscles against your spine, buttocks moving backward as hands and head lead your straight torso forward until it is at a ninety-degree angle to your legs. Swing forward and downward and roll up, finding a nice rhythm.

4. PELVIC TILT

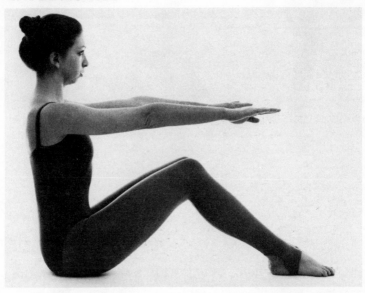

Original Position: Sit on mat, knees bent, feet parallel and in line with hips, standing consciously on the tripod of the foot. Heels are eighteen to twenty-four inches from buttocks. Back is straight. Arms are held out in

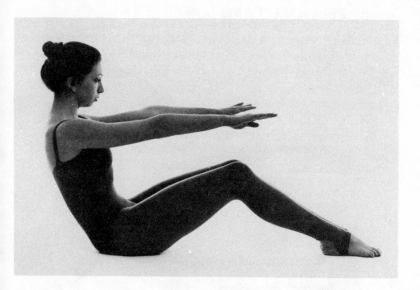

front of you, shoulder width, high and wide, palms down.

Action: Lower vertebrae, one at a time. Coccyx is down, next comes sacrum and then lumbar. Reverse action: Lumbar comes off mat, then the sacrum and end by sitting tall in original position. Inhale first, exhale on lowering. Inhale on rest and exhale coming up.

Objective: Stretch lower spine, thereby strengthening abdominal muscles, breathing comfortably and not involving the shoulder girdle during the action of exercise.

Notes and Comments: Think of tilting pubic bone to chin while lowering vertebrae to mat. Make up an image for yourself, something like: The only way your abdominal muscles can help you will be if they are falling into the cavity of your pelvis and pressing the spine down.

5. PELVIC LIFT AND LOWER

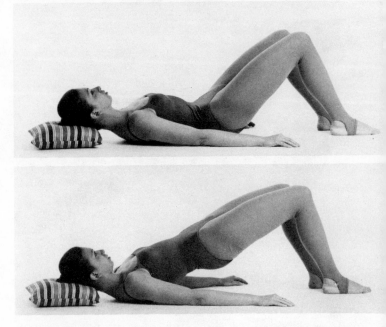

Original Position: Lie on mat or rug with legs bent and feet placed parallel in line with hips, stepping firmly into tripod of foot. Arms are resting comfortably at your sides, palms down.

Action: Inhale before you lift and exhale as you step firmly into your feet, lifting your buttocks high off the floor, *only as high as you can, keeping your abdomen falling into the cavity of your pelvis and your rib cage relaxed.* Inhale while hips are up and exhale as you roll down through your spine, reaching long with your coccyx bone, thinking of putting three inches between each vertebra as you lower your spine.

Objective: To stretch the spine and feel its mobility. In accomplishing this, it is important to keep the buttocks up while trying to touch the small of your back to the mat first. Only when the small of the back reaches the mat are the buttocks lowered.

6. ROLLING THROUGH THE SPINE

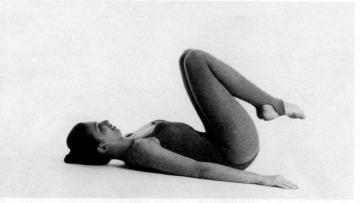

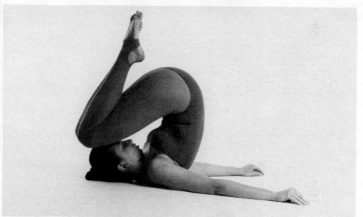

Original Position: Lie on your back on mat or carpet. Hands rest comfortably at your sides with palms down on the mat. Your knees are bent to your chest.

Action: Use your hands pressing into the floor to help you roll your legs over your head. Legs relaxed (knees bent). Roll up to your neck and roll down through the small of the back. Repeat rolling back and forth. Inhale first, exhale rolling up to shoulders, and inhale rolling back to original position.

Objective: Not to hit a flat spot in the spine but to feel it continually rounding.

7. BACK STRAIGHTS

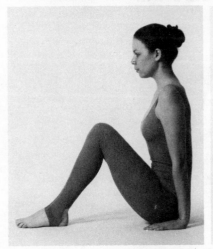
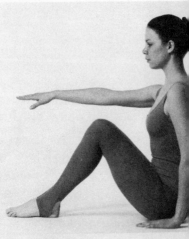

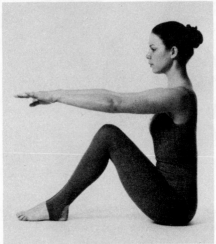

Original Position: Sit up with legs bent and step firmly into the tripod of the feet. Straight arms are in line with your body, palms face down on the floor and fingers facing forward.

Action: Using the back muscles to support the straightness of your back and not lifting with your shoulders, slowly remove one hand as support and hold it straight out in front of you. Then remove the other hand as support and hold it out in front of you.

Objective: To retain a straight back even when your hands are no longer supporting your position.

Notes and Comments: The closer the feet are to the buttocks, the more difficult this exercise becomes.

CHAPTER V

Self-confidence

As I stated previously, my objective in writing this book is to help the reader begin to sense areas in the body which play a prominent part in his or her posture. The exercises given have been carefully chosen to that end. They are a basic set of *awareness movements* to help the performer become acquainted with the flexibility and range of motion of his or her body.

By following this program of structured self-observation (prior to and during the performance of the physical exercises) you will arrive at a time within your own rhythm when you will be able to perform all the physical exercises in this manual, and with these improved perceptions of your body, be qualified to move on to more complicated exercises.

I would like to think of this book as a means of introducing you to your body and hope to awaken in you a desire, not only to improve your posture, but to pursue all the things your new posture will support you in.

Self-confidence and self-knowledge are a marvelously crisscrossing phenomenon—the more self-confident one feels, the more willing one is to learn and the more one learns, the more self-confident one feels. . . . So you see, you can only go forward.